I0845462

Peri, Peri, Quite Contrary

Real Solutions for Perimenopause Weight
Gain, Insomnia, Low Libido and More

Table of Contents

INTRODUCTION

Baptism By Perimenopausal Fire, Why Is Womanhood So Complicated?

I can still remember being almost thirteen years old and wondering why I hadn't gotten my period yet. Sometimes, I feared it might never happen and I'd be stuck in my little girl's body forever, wearing a training bra I didn't even need. Many of my friends bragged about their "monthly visitor." In my mind, they were more mature than I was. More womanly. More sophisticated. More of everything I wanted to be.

But on one unremarkable afternoon, I went to pee, and when I wiped myself, there was a streak of dark red blood!

I panicked. "Mom… I think I need to go to the doctor."

She knocked on the door with a question that embarrassed me in a way that only a mother could. "Sweetie, are you constipated?"

"No!" I snapped as she stepped inside our tiny blue and white bathroom. I held up the toilet paper with a trembling hand, certain it was evidence of a medical catastrophe. "It feels weird. I never had blood…*down there*…before."

She smiled with a hint of pride, revealing dimples which shaved years off her face. Then, she opened a drawer under the sink and handed me a sanitary napkin wrapped in shiny pink plastic. Her words came out in a quick, sing-songy tone, "You just got your first period!"

I was confused. Was this really it? It didn't feel like I expected. To be completely honest, I'd never given serious thought to the sensation of blood shedding from the lining of my uterus. I didn't even know what a uterus was. And back then, the only thing I knew about my vagina was that no one was supposed to touch it except for a doctor.

Mom touched my shoulder. "Every month, this is going to happen. Sometimes, you can tell ahead of time. You might get this feeling in your stomach, you know? But sometimes, it might surprise you. Don't worry, you'll get used to it. You're officially a woman now."

I beamed. This was the moment I'd been anticipating. But before I could revel in the celebration, her smile fell away and her dark eyes narrowed. "But this also means you can get pregnant. Listen to me, you have to be careful. Real, real careful."

As I struggled to take in the gravity of the moment, she showed me how to place the pad in my panties, sticky side down. There were so many random rituals to learn, like wrapping my used sanitary napkins in tissue paper before discarding them in the trash bin. Discretion was a must. It was an initiation to the reality that pieces of the feminine experience had to be hidden. Too unpleasant to show. She also teased that I might want to avoid wearing white for the next few days. And she let me get an extra double-fudge brownie dessert that night, just because.

But my envy for my friends didn't last. Was this womanhood? Having to change pads or tampons every few hours? Cramps that were so debilitating I had to miss school sometimes? Spotting on my favorite pair of jeans?

I asked Mom if this misery would last forever.

She bit her lip and said, "Well, no actually. There's this thing called menopause. It's when a woman stops getting her cycle."

She didn't offer any further explanation at the time, but adolescent me wanted menopause right away! Years later, my wish started to come true in the form of perimenopause. A thing I didn't even know existed until it happened to me. And just like my first period, it wasn't what I expected.

Adult acne. Thinning hair. Being constantly exhausted but unable to sleep. Hot, sweaty nights, even in the dead of winter. A beer belly that rivaled Homer Simpson's. Periods less predictable than airplane departure times. And a sex drive harder to locate than the Bermuda Triangle.

That's perimenopause. "Menopause" *before* menopause. At least that's the way I experienced it. My mother never spoke about it. My aunts were tight-lipped. And my grandmothers? Are you kidding? This whole thing was cloaked in mystery. As a result, I walked around clueless and suffering for a long time.

I'm writing this book because I don't want that to happen to you. I am going to share everything I learned, along with some of my heartbreaking and hilarious misgivings. I will be vulnerable with you and not hold back. Some of this stuff is deeply personal. But if this book can help one woman have an easier time during perimenopause, then it's worth me exposing bizarre and uncomfortable truths about myself.

I'm not a doctor. I'm not a nurse. I'm not a medical professional. I'm not some personal trainer. I'm just a woman who found a way to manage my perimenopause symptoms, and all along the way, I also happened to get into the best shape of my life, experience the best sex in my life and become the best version of myself. All of this *after* the age of forty!

I lost 50 pounds and managed to keep off forty for five years. Okay, that's being honest for you. I'll explain how I gained back 10 if you keep reading. I experienced a sexual awakening that transformed me and the way I look at my body and life in general. I also am finally fulfilled in my career after years of what felt like invisibility.

Take this journey with me. Don't repeat my mistakes. I want you to do more than just cope with the symptoms of perimenopause. Embrace this change of life and even find joy in it. I know that might seem like a stretch right now, but you can get there… One step at a time, one good night's sleep at a time, one goal at a time, and yes, one orgasm at a time too. Let's go!

CHAPTER ONE
Symptoms: Hello, It's Me But It Sure Doesn't Feel Like It

Meet thirty-six-year-old me. On the outside looking in, I seemed to have it "all" and then some. A devoted husband, an adorable 6-year-old son, a full-time job, a four-bedroom house, and a minivan. Family and friends used to shower us with unsolicited commits. "You two are so in love. Wow!" or "You both are amazing parents." or "I don't know how you make it look so easy." I would grin and nod and offer a meek thank you. But there was so much more that I wanted to say.

Beyond the picturesque exterior, I was restless, exhausted, and constantly asking myself, "Is this all there is?" I am not sure how much of what I felt was attributed to perimenopause, the 7-year-itch in my marriage or just an overall hunger for more out of life, but the first thing I can distinctly remember changing was my libido.

When I first met my husband, whom I'll call Carter, there was an instant spark and attraction. From the moment we locked eyes, my desire for him was off the charts. And when we started dating, our first kiss made me tingle in ways that I couldn't even comprehend.

I can remember one very romantic evening where we saw a movie and left the theater as light, fluffy snowflakes fell under the glow of the streetlights. He held my hand and looked deeply into my eyes, and I knew I was already in love. It was a moment worthy of a montage scene in a rom com where the perfect song plays in the background. I knew he was the one. I knew I wanted to marry him.

But fast forward to life with a kid and a ton of bills and meddling in-laws and commuting an hour to work and everything was different. Sex was way at the bottom of the list. I probably gave more thought to dusting the blinds. I just wasn't interested anymore. *At all.*

It wasn't that my husband was unattractive. In all fairness, we'd both packed on a few pounds since saying, "I do." But he was still a handsome man. And it's not that I felt especially self-conscious about the way my body changed after pregnancy. Sure, there were stretch marks and a belly pooch and sagging breasts, but he always assured me with, "You brought our son into the world, you're the most beautiful woman I've ever seen."

But even these words did nothing to reignite my desire. I'd mastered a variety of ways to say "no" without ever saying it. "I have to wake up early tomorrow." "Let me get a raincheck." "Not now, but how about the weekend?" Days would pass, then weeks, sometimes months with no intimacy. We were in a sexless marriage.

He complained about it often, but I was content to remain that way. When I think back on the situation, I'm overcome with sadness. There I was, thirty-six-years-old and giving up on one of the most special things a husband and wife can share. Our dead bedroom put a strain on everything between us. I didn't talk to anyone about it. Who would I have talked to? I didn't bother to get my hormones checked. I just kept existing.

To be completely honest, I wasn't even attracted to other men. I can remember a tall, decent looking guy at work who always went out of his way to synchronize his lunch hour with mine. His eager smile whenever I walked into the break room made his crush on me quite obvious. But I just went about my daily schedule. Indifferent. Unresponsive. Besides, an affair was not something I wanted.

I didn't want anything to do with men. And no, I wasn't attracted to women either. To tell the truth, I didn't even pleasure myself. Gone were the days of taking those tender moments in the shower after a self-breast exam to linger on my nipples and enjoy the sensation of them hardening. And it had been years since I actually masturbated. It was as if the sexual switch inside my body had been shut down completely, like an old computer beyond repair, destined for the cyber junkyard. And the craziest thing about it was that I didn't even care. I didn't miss sex all.

The mediocre compromise I came up with for my husband was performing blow jobs. But even this disappointed him because he wanted nothing more than to please me too. And I wanted nothing more than to not be bothered. We went back and forth and this was a serious point of tension.

Upon further reflection, this was probably the first symptom of perimenopause. I probably should have gotten my hormones tested right away. Yes, thirty-six does seem young, but some of these changes do occur in the mid and late 30's. But a word of warning here, hormonal tests are not completely reliable when it comes to establishing if a woman is in perimenopause. But you should still get the test to rule out thyroid problems or other medical issues. It's also important to trust your instincts and track your symptoms.

I eventually did find a way to restore my sex life. I managed to do so naturally, without prescription meds. I am so grateful that I am no longer neglecting this part of my humanity.

The next big shift I can remember was lack of sleep. I never struggled with this before. As a teenager on Saturday mornings, I slept in until almost eleven o'clock, much to my mother's dismay. "Lazy Bones." That's what she called me.

Years later, when I was in college, staying up late to study for exams or partying all night, I could lay my head on the pillow and fall asleep instantly and slumber away until the annoying buzz of the alarm pierced my ears. Sleep was simple. It's something I gave zero thought to.

In my 20's, I used to unwind with a glass of wine after work. Sometimes two. That relaxing state would always usher me into dreamland. But by the time I hit my mid-30's, sleep was far from easy.

I always went to bed with a long list of worries on my mind. Anxiety about money or the lack thereof. Resentment about being passed over for a promotion at work. Fear that I wasn't putting my son in the right school. Disappointments when I scrolled social media and cross-compared my life to friends from high school. On top of that, I wasn't taking advantage of something that might have relaxed me a bit…making love to my husband.

I'd find myself waking up, usually between two o'clock and three o'clock in the morning, without fail. I went on a mission to fix this. I cut off beverages an hour and a half before bedtime. I took the TV out of the bedroom and avoided looking at my phone before calling it a night. But this didn't seem to help much.

Then, I started down a dangerous road that made things even worse. I went from having a glass of wine or two with dinner to drinking hard liquor right before bed. Rum or whiskey was my favorite go-to. Straight. And like a charm, I fell asleep immediately under the influence, but it never took long before I was up again in the middle of the night and dehydrated too!

My suffering was real. Life without sleep was hell. I didn't know what to do. I was desperate. It took a lot of trial and error before I found a solution that worked for me. These days, I'm waking up well rested and it feels like a slice of heaven!

Some of the other symptoms I felt included having to pee a lot more and occasional incontinence. Every time I went to the grocery store and passed by the adult diaper section, I felt a tinge of embarrassment. I kept pleading with myself, not yet. *Please*, not yet! In general, things were changing down there. I even got some gray pubic hair. Sexy, right? But over time, I did unlock the key to good vaginal health, and I feel much better below the waist and all around.

Gaining weight, especially around the middle, threw me for a loop. I had never been a thin woman. I always considered myself medium to curvy, even before childbirth. But if I was mindful of my calories and exercised, my clothes would fit nicely, and I maintained decent shape. All of a sudden, it was as if my thighs, stomach, hips, and butt were stroked with a fattening paintbrush. One piece of birthday cake and I practically needed a larger dress size! And don't even get me started on bread.

When I was much younger, I remember going out to dinner with women in their forty's and 50's and watching them as they ordered salads with vinaigrette dressing on the side and said no thanks to Cheddar Bay Biscuits at Red Lobster.

I used to say, "Come on, why don't you live a little?" But now that I'm on the other side of that equation I understand their choices.

Still, I refused to be a person who couldn't enjoy amazing food and the occasional dessert or glass of wine. And the thought of counting calories for the rest of my days was less than appealing surgery without anesthesia. There had to be another way. I eventually figured it out and I look forward to sharing that with you.

Let's be honest, perimenopause is a punch to the guts, more accurately, it's a punch to the hormones. But I learned how to put on my boxing gloves and step into the ring. There is a pathway to being the champion of your own health when it comes to this big life change. The first and most important step is to identify if this is what's happening to you.

Here is a checklist of all my own symptoms that I tracked:
1. Frequent urination
2. Going to sleep just fine but waking up in the middle of the night randomly and having trouble falling back to sleep

3.   Lighter periods for fewer days sometimes

4.   Heavier periods with lots of clots sometimes

5.   Irritability

6.   Weight gain

7.   Vaginal dryness

8.   No interest in sex

9.   Thinning hair

10.   Heart palpitations

11.   Hairs on my chin (three to be exact)

12.   Back fat (more than usual)

It took two years before I finally went to the doctor with this list. I had done extensive online research and I was sure that I was in perimenopause. He listened to the thirty-eight-year-old me describe all these changes and pushed his wire-frame glasses up on the bridge of his narrow nose. "I think it's just stress. You're much too young for perimenopause. And vaginal dryness? A woman your age shouldn't have that. No way."

I felt dismissed and devastated. But after a little more conversation, he reluctantly agreed to draw blood for my hormonal tests. I waited weeks and weeks. And finally, when the results were in, I was shocked to see that all my hormonal levels were completely normal. *What?!*

According to the only medical tests that were available at the time, I was not in perimenopause. But my thyroid levels were normal. So was my liver and everything else. How could the test be wrong? My body was not lying to me. So despite his non-diagnosis, I knew what was happening and I went on a journey to heal myself. Here's what happened…

CHAPTER TWO
Coping With Stress: From Screams To Smiles And Everything Between

A few weeks before Christmas, at the age of thirty-eight, I thought I was having a stroke. I can distinctly remember getting out of bed that morning and rushing to the kitchen for coffee. I was functioning on 45 minutes of sleep as I reached for my "BEST MOM" mug.

That first cup of black gold didn't quite do it. But the second cup helped get me in gear and I knew there would be a fresh pot waiting for me as soon as I got to work. I hurried to shower and put on some makeup in an attempt to disguise my ragged under eye circles. I threw some slacks, a sweater, and a pair of flat shoes that I wouldn't have been caught dead in ten years earlier.

On the drive to work, there was traffic. Much more than usual. And I had a headache that was flirting with migraine status. I turned up the music and reached for my water bottle, convinced I was merely dehydrated. Too much coffee, I thought. I had pledged to cut back, but then again, there was a long list of pledges and promises I'd broken to myself.

Then, it happened. The muscles on the left side of my face tightened up and my eye started twitching. I was in denial. Did that just happen? I guzzled down some water and took several deep breaths. Whatever it was, I hoped it was over. Like an idiot, I kept driving.

At the stoplight, it hit me again. This time, the sensation was much stronger. My heart raced as I dared to glance at my reflection in the driver's side mirror. The left side of my face twisted up all over again. *Oh God*, I thought as I finally had enough sense to pull over and park my car in front of a seven-day dry cleaners on a busy avenue.

I called the nurse advice line on the back of my health insurance card and spoke the words out loud in disbelief, "I think… I think I'm having a stroke." Tears rushed down my face as I described my symptoms to a woman with a bristly southern drawl. "Ma'am, from everything you're describing, you need to get to a doctor right away."

Thirty-eight did seem young to have a stroke. But a few years earlier, a friend of mine whom I'll call Nicole, came over to visit me. I hadn't seen her for a while, and I was looking forward to catching up. She was a gorgeous, thin woman of only thirty-two. Model thin. The kind that only comes via genetics.

Over iced tea and my homemade macadamia cookies, we swapped stories about parenthood. As I was refilling her glass, she blurted out, "I'm really trying to pace myself… It's soccer practice on Mondays and Wednesdays and dance lessons on Saturdays. I look up on Sunday and it's like, 'Where did the week go?' But I make it a point to squeeze in a walk every day. Even if it's just ten minutes. And I barely have time for that, but I still do it 'cause I'm not trying to have another stroke, you know."

I stared at her, wondering if I'd misheard something. "You had a stroke?"

She took a deep breath and nodded. "Yeah. It was seven months ago."

I wrapped my arms around her. "Why didn't you tell me? Are you alright?" She described in detail how the stresses of her job, single motherhood, and anxiety about making the mortgage converged on her all at once. It happened right in her cubicle on an ordinary Thursday morning. She felt this sensation on the left side of her body and was rushed to the emergency room. Thankfully, she made a full recovery, but her story always stayed with me.

I always pictured stroke victims as people over the age of seventy with a myriad of health complications. But Nicole? If it could happen to her, then no one was immune. And definitely not me.

As the telehealth nurse encouraged me to calm down and take deep breaths, I feared all the things that could happen, from paralysis to memory lost. When I was finally face-to-face with a petite young doctor in a white lab coat, she told me that my blood pressure was dangerously high and that I probably needed medication to control it. But I was relieved to discover that it wasn't a stroke. It was an anxiety attack.

An anxiety attack? *What?!* How in the world could anxiety cause what happened to me? It didn't make sense. She wrote me some prescriptions for meds I couldn't pronounce. When I went to the pharmacy to get them filled, it dawned on me that maybe I didn't need the pills. Maybe I just needed to change my whole life.

What I didn't tell the doctor was that I knew the source of my anxiety and it went deeper than perimenopause. My marriage was a mess. I hadn't been happy at my job for years. The only real bright spot in my life was my son. Other than that, I felt like a shell of a woman, like everything that made me feel like "me" had been hollowed out.

I'd been in therapy at the time for over a year. Eventually, Carter joined me in therapy too. There was a lot to unpack, but to be completely honest, by the time we started therapy our relationship was on life support.

There were several issues that led to the demise of what we shared. As I reflect on it now, the biggest challenge for me was that what I needed in a partner changed drastically. Although I loved Carter, I began to dread growing old with him.

I was a constant worrier with a special talent for conjuring the worst outcomes for every situation. When my mother wasn't calling me "Lazy Bones", "Worry Wart" was her other nickname for yours truly. When I lived on my own, I faithfully paid my rent early in the form of a cashier's check. Before I got married, I never missed a birth control pill and always made my boyfriend wear a condom. And I still treat yellow lights like red lights.

But in the way that opposites attract, I ended up falling for Carter. His easy-going approach to life was exciting at first. Every day was an adventure for him. He never stressed about finances and just quit jobs on whim if he felt like it, convinced there was always something better out there.

We started off in a modest apartment, romancing each other with cheap home cooked meals and I was over the moon. Carter was sweet and sensual and everything I thought I wanted in a man. Happiness overflowed like the bowls of pasta we loved to indulge in.

But after I gave birth to our son, Carter's free spirit no longer meshed with the cost of diapers and daycare. Our finances were so strained that I found myself going to foodbanks to make ends meet. On top of that, he *could not* or *would not* keep a job for long. So I always was the one working full-time, sometimes I worked two jobs.

Long before perimenopause, the whole situation made my vagina dry up like the Sahara Desert. When I looked at Carter, I didn't see a man who wanted to provide for me and our son. I saw an entitled little boy in a grown man's body. He was content to let me figure out a way to keep our family from drowning, no matter how much it exhausted me.

I didn't talk to anyone about this except for my therapist. I was embarrassed. It made me feel less than worthy. When I looked around, I saw men in my family who worked hard and took care of their wives. And I resented not having that myself.

The onset of perimenopause illuminated all these feelings. I remember one day when I was in the backyard, pulling up a weed and Carter rushed over to me. He knew I was on edge because we were two months late on our electricity bill and probably on the verge of a shutoff notice.

He kneeled to kiss my sweaty cheek. "Don't worry, I took care of it."

I smiled and thanked him. But before I could breathe a sigh of relief, he added, "I just put it on the credit card, so we're good." I wanted to punch the sky. As he walked back into the house with his nonchalant stride, I thought to myself, *What's going to happen when I'm fifty years old? I can't go on like this.*

I grew up comfortably middle class. Some of my friends might even say I was spoiled. There might be some truth to that. Because my father was a successful entrepreneur, I had access to a world of unique experiences at an early age. On some of his business trips, he would bring us along and we went all around the country, and on occasion, there was international travel too.

But fast forward to my married life with Carter and there I was, in a small backyard of a rented house, sitting in the dirt of what was supposed to be a beautiful garden. I thought about all sorts of things like the fact that Carter and I hadn't even been on a date in five months. There was no money for that, of course. I looked down at the weed in my hands and wanted to cry. This was right before my anxiety attack.

The day I went home with those prescription pills, I told Carter, "I need to make some changes in my life, so this never happens again." He nodded, seeming to understand. But what was in the forefront of my mind was the knowledge that if things didn't get better, I could no longer stay in the marriage. My health was at stake.

Right then and there, I stopped breaking promises to myself. I thought of Nicole as I took a walk in the neighborhood park after work. I would put on my earbuds and listen to a podcast or my favorite songs. Sometimes, I only had twenty minutes. On the weekends, I was out there for a whole hour. The fresh air and sunshine made me feel brand new. And on the cold days, I bundled up and walked around the block a time or two just to stay in the habit.

When it came to Carter, I made my feelings known. The unfiltered version of me angered him. We got into more arguments than ever before. But despite this, I felt much better. I was no longer crying into my pillow hoping he would just miraculously figure out how to improve our marriage. Instead, I was letting it all out with the occasional four-letter word.

Another big change I made was carving out more quality time with our son. Between taking him back and forth to school and playdates and getting him off to basketball practice, I felt like more of a shuttle service than a mother sometimes. So I made it a point for us to do other things together like make homemade pizzas, paint pictures and read classics books.

As for things at my job, I ended up getting laid off because the company was relocating out of state. Before I even had time to panic about money, a job I had applied to a year earlier contacted me about an opening. It paid less but it also had more schedule flexibility. I was so grateful for the timing of it all.

I also started to keep a journal. I wasn't always consistent with my entries, I mostly wrote whenever my stress was at a fever pitch. I often cried during this process. But it was very helpful.

I kept seeing my therapist. Having someone to talk to that wasn't a friend or family member made me feel like I wasn't judged for my true emotions. These sessions usually evoked tears, but just like the journaling, I always felt more at peace afterwards.

Meanwhile, things got so bad between me and Carter that we ended up sleeping in separate rooms. The biggest upside to this was that I did get a better night's sleep. But there were obvious disadvantages, especially as our son began to ask more questions.

I don't have any regrets in my life. Every moment helped to shape the woman I am. But if I was to give advice to a younger version of myself, I would emphasize the importance of thinking beyond the here and now. If I'm being completely honest with myself, the twenty-something-year-old me wanted someone cute and fun and great in bed. But the forty-something-year-old me craved a man who took joy in being a provider and making sure I was okay. Carter had never really been that guy, but was there any possibility of him changing?

I came to find out that I wasn't the only one going through this. As women age, our needs and our hormones evolve. We are biologically wired to require different levels of support and we shouldn't feel any shame in admitting that. So, for any younger women reading this, please take heed!

Checklist for Coping With Stress & Anxiety:

1.   **What is really bugging you?** Ask yourself this difficult question. It might be several things, but chances are, there is one thing that truly stands out above the rest. The thing you find yourself thinking about several times a day. Name and identify it. In my experience, perimenopause shines an even brighter light on whatever challenges you're facing.

2.   **Write it down**. Share your unfiltered self on the page. Even if you keep an old-fashioned journal under literal lock and key, this can be so liberating. You can

feel free to describe people and situations in whatever colorful language you choose, and you might even find yourself laughing after the tears.

3.   **See a doctor.** Don't wait until you're driving to work with an anxiety attack like I did. When something feels off, go get checked out. And stay consistent with appointments. Oftentimes as women, we are overseeing the medical care of kids, parents and loved ones while completely passing ourselves over. Stop that. Today!

4.   **Be honest with the people you love.** Many of us mask our feelings behind responses like, "I'm fine," knowing good and damn well that we are far from it. Whether you need to have a heart-to-heart with your partner, child, co-worker, or friend, don't hold back. Keeping it inside only harms you. And if they shut down and refuse to listen then that speaks volumes about their lack of love and empathy for you. But you should love yourself enough not to put up with crap from anyone, never mind their temper tantrums.

5.   **Walk every day.** I know it's not easy to make time for this and depending on the weather, it can be tricky, but carve out at least ten minutes for this. I used to do this on my lunch break, ten minutes to eat and twenty minutes to walk. I always came back to the desk more refreshed and ready to tackle the second half of the day.

6.   **Identify what you need to change.** If your marriage isn't working or your job isn't fulfilling, analyze what you want to be different and make an action plan

to get there. There might be small things you can do, like plan a special date night or go to a job fair. Eventually, you can work towards bigger goals but try to do something every week to address this.

7.   **Therapy can help.** A good counselor is a treasure. A bad one is a disaster. Sometimes, you might have to try a few before finding the right fit… It's kind of like shopping for clothes. Don't give up. Your mental health is too important to neglect. And a good counselor will give you tools to cope between sessions that make your day-to-day existence less chaotic.

8.   **Build on what brings you joy.** Carve out more time for the people and things you really love. Even if it's just an extra phone call or video chat a week with your best friend to say "hi", it is going to make you feel so much better. A few laughs with your favorite cousin might just add years to your life.

9.   **Treat yourself.** Even if it's something simple like a bowl of strawberries or a facial, you deserve to do something nice for you. And only you! Once a month is the bare minimum, so please start there. For me, I love to get pedi while I power up the massage chair. It's thirty minutes of bliss followed by a trip to the grocery store across the street for some gourmet cheese to enjoy with a glass of wine at home.

10.   **Give yourself grace.** Some days are gonna be rough. And that's okay. Hit the reset button tomorrow. And if tomorrow turns out to be trash, there's always the day after tomorrow. Roll those lessons over as you keep getting closer to the peace your heart longs for.

11.   A word about prayer. If you believe in a Higher Power, as I do, then take time to pray. I pray throughout the day… I have lots of little conversations with God and it always lifts my spirits. If you don't believe in a Higher Power, tap into meditation. These quiet moments are critical for stress management and so much more.

After doing these things, my blood pressure returned to the normal range without medication, and I didn't suffer from further anxiety attacks. But this was just my experience. I am not advocating against prescription meds. I asked my doctor for permission to try to improve on my own first before starting the pills and she agreed. I was very intentional about monitoring my blood pressure at home with the understanding that I might still need to start taking them. So far, I haven't had to but who knows what the future will bring? All I know for certain is that the fear of having a stroke in my 30's was a glaring reminder that I'm no good to anyone if I don't take care of myself first.

CHAPTER THREE
Insomnia, Amber Alert! Sound Sleep
Has Gone Missing!

The moment I held my newborn son in my arms, he looked up at me with those bright, beady little eyes. His drooling mouth curled into the sweetest, toothless smile. I felt love so pure and perfect that I couldn't help but cry. He would change my life forever in unexpected and wonderful ways. He would also change my sleep forever too. For the sake of this book, I'll call him Justin.

The very first night I came home from the hospital, my son woke up five times to nurse! As a first-time mother, my virgin nipples were unprepared for the pulling, tugging, and sucking that ensued. And when the morning came, I felt fatigued like never before.

My mother came over on her way to work to watch him while I took a bath. When I submerged my sore body into the warm water, a sense of calm came over me as I closed my eyes. Moments later, she banged on the door like law enforcement serving a warrant. "Hurry up, I'm gonna be late."

I quickly soaped up my weary body and stepped out of a

bubbly oasis onto the cold, tiled floor. I wrapped myself in a towel, my belly still swollen from childbirth, I probably looked about seven months pregnant. When I opened the bathroom door, Mom stood there, holding little Justin who didn't look so cute anymore because his tiny face was red from bawling. She handed him to me and said, "Umph. That sounds like a hungry cry."

"Mom, I'm tired. I didn't get any sleep last night and–"

"You've got some nerve, complaining. Could be worse. Imagine what I went through, getting pregnant back-to-back. I didn't get a good night's sleep for over two years, girlie."

"But–"

"Welcome to motherhood. Don't forget to burp him good after he finishes eating. We wouldn't want my sweet little grandson getting gas. Can't have that." She playfully tickled his feet and rushed out the door.

Women from my mother's generation never complained. They pushed through their problems and kept up appearances. They spoke among their friends in brave tones about all they endured. It was a sort of Olympics of misery, usually topped off with a phrase like, "Young mothers have it so much easier now-a-days."

But the fact that Mom was indifferent to my insomnia didn't make it any less real. I looked at little Justin in my arms. How could something so precious take a hacksaw to any chance at decent sleep?

Eight months later, I can distinctly remember the first time he slept through the night. I got six hours of rest, and I woke up and planted kisses all over his head of curls. "Thanks for letting Mommy sleep. I love you so much!"

Years later, at the age of thirty-seven, I found myself fighting insomnia all over again, but this time it had nothing to do with Justin. Every night, I went to bed and drifted off to sleep. Without fail, I would be suddenly awake at some ungodly hour between two and three o'clock in the morning.

I looked over at the alarm clock in misery… It was way too early to wake up. I'd toss and turn and change positions, desperate to get back to dreamland. Most of the time, this never worked. On the rare occasion I did fall back asleep, it would always be within a few minutes of having to get out of bed and start my day.

I read once that operating without adequate sleep is akin to drunkenness. Well, coffee was the antidote for that, at least that's what I thought as I hustled my butt into the kitchen every morning for that fix. I couldn't help but laugh to myself at the thought that I used to drink coffee socially in my 20's. Now, it was an everyday thing, and on the weekdays, there was usually more than one cup.

Back then, I did not know that insomnia was a symptom of perimenopause. I didn't know anything about perimenopause. And the only thing I knew about menopause at that time was what I saw in pharmaceutical commercials where women described hot flashes. At this point, my mother had already experienced all these things, but she never opened up to me except to say, "It wasn't so bad as most women make it out to be."

As I reflect on her words now, I can't help but think that she was most likely downplaying the realities of how difficult the transition was. Much like the day she came over to watch Justin and could not empathize with my delirious state after a very restless night with a newborn.

It took a few years before I embraced the reality of being in perimenopause. Doctors and hormonal tests be damned! My body wasn't lying to me. That constant waking up in the middle of the night…even when I didn't have to pee, there was clearly something going on. And unlike my mother's generation, I had no desire to compete in the misery Olympics.

I was determined to find a way to get a good night's sleep again. One day, my father came to visit and gifted me a bottle of top shelf whiskey. When I went into the kitchen to make him a drink, I asked him if he wanted ice or soda. He replied, "No, I'll have it straight."

"Really?"

"Yeah. It's better that way and I drink less. Just an ounce or two in the glass is all I need."

"Okay, I'll try that too."

We toasted with two whiskeys. Neat. No chaser. No ice. It was a smooth, mellow feeling. That night, I got the best sleep I'd had in a long time. I thought it was because of the whiskey. In all actuality, it was probably my dad's crazy stories that brought on belly laughs.

The next night, I helped myself to a shot of whiskey alone. I woke up again in the middle of the night. My mouth was so dry that I felt the sensation to cough. I rushed to get water. I tried to go back to sleep and that was impossible. A slight headache was coming on as I rustled in bed. The suffering was real.

I decided to try sober January. As a longtime lover of wine and the occasional stiff drink, I looked forward to seeing what it felt like to quit alcohol altogether. I had more energy and my skin looked better, but good sleep was still a distant stranger.

I read online about the benefits of melatonin and decided to try it. I thought it was safe, a vitamin that you can buy at most pharmacies. Harmless, right? Immediately, I started to sleep better, but over time, the effects faded. I discovered that if I increased my dose from one pill to two pills that I was back in business, but soon my body became accustomed to that too. I feared I might become dependent on melatonin, and I refused to take three pills, so I stopped altogether.

My insomnia came back worse than before. I did a little research and came across the benefits of medical marijuana in the form of edibles. I had never been a weed smoker. I absolutely hated the smell and all of the stoners I knew in high school and college were not exactly poster children for "Most Likely To Succeed." I steered clear off the stuff and stuck to just one vice…alcohol, wine in particular.

It's laughable when I think about it now, but the first time I got high I was almost thirty-eight years old. I ate half of an edible oatmeal cookie and it took me into another stratosphere. For some people, marijuana can cause paranoia. That didn't happen to me, but I do remember looking at some silly movie on TV and laughing so hard I could barely control my bladder. And I was super relaxed, my mind worry free in a way that almost terrified me. That night, I slept harder than I had since my teenage years.

But much like melatonin, I did not want to become dependent on edibles. I felt like it was fine to have them once in a while, but I didn't want to turn into the kind of person who felt the need to get high every day. So, I continued to search for different sleep solutions.

I made the choice to cut back on alcohol. I limit myself to a glass and a half a day, no more than two. Sometimes, I don't have any. This helped me feel more in control of myself and my life in general and did help my sleep. And while I still enjoy hard liquor, I will mix it with tea or tonic water so I'm not dehydrated.

Another big change was to eat dinner earlier. There were times when I had to work late and didn't get home until nine o'clock. Putting a heavy dinner on my stomach and then crashing was a disaster. Perimenopause or not, I had to make some changes. On days I worked late, I ate dinner at work so when I got home, I could unwind and get ready for bed.

As cruel as this may sound, sleeping in a separate room from my husband helped too. Carter always came to bed after me. If I was in bed by ten o'clock, he'd climb into the sheets about an hour and half later, disrupting the start of whatever potential sleep I had. On top of that, he snored too. And even worse, when he was angry, he'd keep me up with rants about all his grievances. But by this point, I already had one foot out the door and I was just desperate to protect my sanity and peace.

I also exercised more. I'd never been a gym rat, but I did find that being more active helped me sleep better. And there was no way I would give up desserts, but I avoided having them late at night. It's so much easier on your digestive system to have the apple pie earlier in the afternoon instead of thirty minutes before bedtime.

I also stopped drinking everything an hour and half before going to sleep. I have a routine that relaxes me when I lay down which includes reading or listening to music but no TV and no phone. And I always end each day with a prayer and reflection of what I'm grateful for.

Checklist for a better night's sleep:

1.   **Don't eat late.** I know this is hard sometimes but try to stop eating at least two hours before you call it a night. I struggled with this, but it made a big difference when I became more intentional about planning out my dinner times. And on the days I eat late, I will stay awake later.

2.   **Don't drink late.** This goes for alcohol, water, and everything else. I don't drink an hour and a half before bedtime. I treat myself like a giant toddler. This also reduces that terrible sensation of waking up in the middle of the night to have to pee.

3.   **Eat junk food earlier.** There is no way I would give up French fries or cupcakes. Perimenopause be damned! But I try not to eat any of this stuff four hours before bedtime. When those late-night cravings come over me, I reach for strawberries or blueberries. Then, I wait ten minutes and decide if it's worth it to stuff my face with chocolate. 99% of the time the answer is hell no. Sweet and salty food is harder to digest and I treasure sleeping too much to risk it.

4.   **Get moving.** Going for walks is great. But the best sleep I got was after I joined my local YMCA and went swimming! Wow, something about being in the water really relaxed my whole body. The most important thing is to do something every day and challenge

yourself to do more incrementally.

5.   Melatonin can help. There are many benefits to this. If you're really suffering, then by all means, try it for a month or two. But it's important to monitor your usage. I was very close to developing a dependency even though it is supposedly non addictive. Everyone is different so your experience may not mirror my own.

6.   Enjoy edibles. If you are open-minded to using marijuana, it might be helpful but please do yourself a favor and start small. For example, try one gummy and then wait an hour or an hour and a half before reaching for a second one. You might find you don't need it or want it. The body high that edibles bring can be very strong. One time, I was so high that it carried over until the morning and I wasn't able to be fully present for my son. "Mommy, why are your eyes so red?" Don't let that be you!

7.   Sleep alone. This is not always an option. But if it is possible, you might find that a bed by yourself could be just the fix you need. If you share a bed with a partner and have to deal with another human's bodily functions and deep breathing on top of your insomnia, it can drive you crazy. This is especially true if you're having a rough patch in your relationship like I was.

8.   Make a bedtime routine. Take a warm bath and listen to some music. Read a chapter of a book. Masturbate! Do whatever it takes to help you unwind before going to sleep. If you are consistent, it will help to retrain your body to start shutting down.

9.   Drink less coffee. If you can't cut back, don't

touch it after lunchtime. This also should apply to caffeinated sodas and energy drinks. Many of us need that afternoon cup to power through the rest of the day, I understand from experience. But try green tea or non-sugary alternatives instead.

10. **White noise and other colors may help.** You may decide to purchase a white noise machine or even try an app on your phone. Apparently, there are several varieties of this calming noise including brown noise, blue noise and pink noise. I even use these when I travel to feel more relaxed in strange bed and it works surprisingly well.

11. **When you wake up in the middle of the night…** Even if you do everything "right", it still happens. Have some go-to's to help you get back to sleep. It might be deep breathing or meditation. It might be a self-massage. Worst case scenario, you might have to get out of bed to do something until you're drowsy again. Avoid TV. Read a boring book. But not this one, I hope.

When I started to do these things, sleep became much easier. I still have the occasional restless night but it's much more manageable. In the previous chapter, I highlighted tools for reducing stress. All these things worked in tandem to help me get beauty rest. And one of the side benefits I didn't expect was that my under eye circles are practically gone!

CHAPTER FOUR
Weight Gain: The Double Chin
And The Double Chocolate

At work one day, I felt a sharp pain shoot through my back. I was on the verge of tears as I begged for permission to leave early. I drove home in a daze and limped through my front door. I scrambled for the Tylenol and drank a ton of water. Then, I climbed into bed and twisted myself into odd shapes, desperate for relief. I hoped that I'd be back to normal with the rising sun.

But the next morning, my burning ache had only intensified. As I reached for the phone on the nightstand, I hollered like an old woman in a "Life Alert" commercial. I took several deep breaths and called my boss.

"Hey...um... I don't think I can make it in, my back is still killing me."

"But you I let you go home early yesterday—"

"I know, but—"

"What did your doctor tell you?"

"I didn't go in yet, I just came straight home...to try to sleep it off..."

My supervisor sighed. "I need to see a note from a physician or else I can't pay you for today. Are we clear?"

I hung up and drove myself straight to urgent care. At every stoplight, I shifted my butt around in my seat like a teenager trying to go viral with a new dance. But I was even more concerned about the status of my employment than my back. I crossed my fingers I'd get prescribed meds strong enough to help me power through the rest of the workday. I even sent a text to my boss that read: "About to see the doctor now, hope to be back in the office asap :)"

Under the lobby's fluorescent lights, I fumbled with a pen and a stack of forms on a clipboard, demanding endless facts about my medical history followed by a questionnaire about my cat. Okay. That's a slight exaggeration, but I was spent. By the time I filled everything out, I thought I might pass out in that ugly orange chair, across from a rack of glossy health magazines.

The nurse finally called my name and escorted me to a room where he took my blood pressure. It was a relief to see that it was in the normal range. Then, he asked me to step on the scale. The number I saw took my breath away. 184 pounds. My heart raced. That was the biggest I'd ever been. I was even larger than I was in the ninth month of my pregnancy.

I went from worrying about my back to panicking about my size. How *and* when did I get here? I waited in a sterile white patient room, looking at a diagram of human organs. I thought about how my own must be surrounded by fat. Swimming in it. Drowning in it.

I was confused. I hadn't changed my diet or exercise habits lately. Sure, I wasn't the world's most health-conscious woman but I still made an effort. Back then, I cooked a majority of my meals and walked at least three times a week.

I wasn't always consistent but what else was new? In the past, when I packed on the pounds, I always could point to a culprit like Halloween candy or my aunt's southern fried cooking on summer vacation.

This time, I came up blank. I thought I was healthy. And although I'd never viewed myself as "thin", I'd never considered myself fat either. A solid medium build. That was me. But clearly not anymore.

Eventually, I would find out that perimenopause played a big role in this. Of course, I was clueless about it at the time. All I felt was shame. How could I let myself go like that? As a child, I often wondered why middle aged women tended to be heavy. The answer was probably a combination of hormonal changes, stressful lifestyles and weight from childbirth that never completely went away.

At that moment, I realized that I was one of them… One of those overweight women pushing shopping carts down superstore aisles in shapeless sweatpants. If I'm being completely honest, I had at least three pairs of them at home with stretched-out waistbands.

The doctor tapped on the door. "May I come in?"

I battled my oncoming tears. "Mmmhmmm."

"Sorry, I couldn't hear you."

"Ah...yeah. I said yeah."

She walked inside. A petite woman with a short asymmetrical haircut, glasses, and a narrow forehead. She looked fresh out of med school. Her arched eyebrows furrowed.

"I understand you're experiencing back pain. When did

this start?"

"Yesterday. It...it just came out of nowhere. I was at work and...it just...pow!"

"Is your job strenuous?"

"Not exactly, I sit at a desk all day."

She scribbled some notes on her pad.

"I'm going to prescribe you a muscle relaxer and something else to help with the pain."

"Okay. Thanks. I appreciate that. I never knew my back could hurt so bad. Do you know what caused it?"

"It's hard to pinpoint, but I hope you won't be offended when I say that these sorts of pains can be exacerbated by excess pounds."

I swallowed and nodded. "I know I'm a little heavy. I couldn't believe what I saw on the scale today."

"To be honest, you're not overweight."

"Really?" I smiled a little. Okay. Maybe it wasn't as bad as I thought. My body relaxed. Suddenly, my back felt better too. I figured I was being too hard on myself. A habit that had only worsened with age.

"You're not overweight because you're technically obese."

Wait. *What?! Obese?* I thought of how I'd been buying larger pant sizes in the past few months. I reasoned with myself that I hadn't actually gained weight, but blamed the manufacturers instead. Every designer made clothes differently, right?

But with the doctor peering at me through her designer glasses, the truth hung in the air like a foul stench, immune to a hundred scented candles. I. Was. Obese. And I had been in denial about it up until that moment.

"I really hope you take better care of yourself. I've seen patients begin a slow creep...to 200 pounds...then 250 and so on. It can be a slippery slope, putting you at higher risk for hypertension, diabetes, high cholesterol, and morbid obesity..."

Her words trailed off. I imagined my body expanding, like a hot air balloon until it just exploded. Like the girl who smacked too much blueberry chewing gum in "Willy Wonka and the Chocolate Factory."

On the drive home, I passed by my favorite fried fish restaurant and willed myself to keep on driving. I grabbed a grilled salmon and vegetable dish for lunch and water instead. I fought back my craving for candy-sweet strawberry lemonade. I was determined to start making changes immediately.

That day, I went for a very long walk in a neighborhood with plenty of hills. Despite the autumn's cool air, I worked up a sweat as I hustled up inclines, using muscles that had been dormant for ages. At the end of my walk, I promised myself that I was going to be more consistent with exercise. The thought of poking myself with needles to check my blood sugar daily like my grandmother sent chills through me.

I did not think there was anything wrong with my diet before, but I read that most people have no idea how much they eat until they track it. I downloaded a free app to get a handle on things. I was amazed at what it revealed.

For breakfast, I liked coffee with almond milk and sugar, a tall glass of orange juice and a bowl of cereal which I assumed was healthy. For lunch, I usually ate something on the go, like a tuna melt sandwich and fries from the restaurant across the street from my job. For dinner, spaghetti or chicken with rice were my go-tos. And I loved to top off the day with two or three brownies and wine or a mixed drink. Much like the famous song, I did love pina coladas!

After a few days of tracking my meals, I was shocked to see how much sugar was in the so-called "healthy foods" I ate. My morning cereal had more sugar than the brownies I indulged in. A glass of my favorite lemonade was the sugar equivalent of three cookies. And don't even get me started on a pina colada!

I decided that cutting back on added sugars was a must, but instead of giving up everything sweet, I started with drinks. Instead of orange juice, I ate real fruit. Instead of lemonade, I drank water or unsweetened iced tea. And I still ate brownies but made sure not to get carried away. And most nights, my dessert consisted of strawberries and chocolate covered almonds. I swapped out pina coladas for dry red wine.

I knew I didn't want to do any crazy diets. My friends who were on Keto all turned into rabid animals when they were within the vicinity of ice cream or potatoes. I needed something I could stick with long term.

I took the same approach when it came to exercise. I didn't join a gym and start a crazy, unsustainable regime. I never really liked gyms to be honest. The sweaty people, the occasional creepy man staring at me like I was on a stripper pole, not to mention the fit women who made me feel self-conscious, intentional or not.

I figured walking would be the easiest thing and it was something I already enjoyed. I committed to doing a lap in the neighborhood park every day. And on the weekends, I walked twice a day.

When it came to cooking, I swapped white rice for brown

rice. I also used extra virgin olive oil instead of butter. And I also ate dinner earlier. Sometimes as early as five o'clock if I could swing it.

I also was intentional about getting back in touch with my sexuality. Although things were so strained between me and Carter that intimacy was not on the radar, I decided that shouldn't stop me. For the first time in years, I masturbated. The orgasmic explosion courtesy of my fingers made my body tingle with ecstasy and literally wiped away all my stress!

I also observed my body in the mirror with gratitude every day. Naked. I took in my pot belly, love handles, cellulite and stretch marks too. But I made it a point to see past the shell of my exterior and give thanks for my life and the fact that my body had been a vessel to bring my son into the world.

I didn't obsess over the scale. I kept my weigh-ins to once a week or every other week. It was a slow, steady journey to get healthier. Eventually, almost a year later, I'd lost 50 pounds. I couldn't believe it!

There were times when I would gain back some weight. I soon found myself under-eating and overdoing it with cardio. That was just as dangerous as my obesity had been. My body hungered for a healthy balance.

Strength training was the game changer I needed. I also started to eat more protein. And I stopped depriving myself too. I made sure I ate enough every day, especially plenty of fruits and vegetables. And if I felt like a cookie, I helped my-self.

Eventually, I gained back 10 pounds. Most of it was mus-cle. Muscle weighs more than fat, so I didn't really care about the number on the scale. But I noticed with more muscle tone, my clothes fit better and I had even more energy. I also found that lifting weights helped me feel stronger.

Five years later, I am still going strong on my fitness journey. I came to appreciate my progress with gratitude. Perimenopause causes hormonal swings in women that make much fat harder to burn.

But one recurring theme you've probably picked up so far is that I had a bad habit of waiting until my body broke down to finally make changes. Between my anxiety attack that I feared was a stroke and my excruciating back pain, I had a pattern of neglecting myself until it was almost too late.

While it's important to maintain a healthy weight, it's far more important to listen to your body when it's trying to communicate, no matter what your size. And it's also crucial to love your body, no matter what your size. In a society that nods and winks at "dad bods" and expects women to maintain bikini bodies, it's difficult but necessary to maintain your sense of self. But you must!

<u>Checklist for getting to and maintaining a healthy weight:</u>

1.   **Listen to your body.** It is actually trying to talk to you if you shut your big mouth and really listen! For some people, getting healthier means a complete fitness overall like I did. For others, it might mean just exercising more and losing five or ten pounds. Find your body's natural happy place.

2.   **Don't overdo it.** Too much cardio and not eating enough can actually backfire on weight loss goals. Not to mention if you're anything like me, you're a night-

mare to be around when you're hungry. So take heed!

3. **Pile up on protein.** I like a combination of plant-based protein like almonds combined with chicken breasts, salmon and occasionally beef. I also love non-fat Greek yogurt which helps keep me regular too. Not to gross you out, but fiber is a very big part of the picture. You might not even be overweight; you might just be bloated and constipated.

4. **Replace as many drinks as possible with water.** I give myself a bit of variety by putting fresh fruit in my water for flavor or dropping in a delicious bag of tea. I also drink water in between glasses of wine. More water will help you stay healthy and for me, it also made my skin look years younger. Sometimes, I wonder how much dehydration had to do with some of my previous health problems.

5. **Strength training is your friend.** I walk every day because it relaxes me and helps me stay active but the key to losing weight and sculpting my body was picking up some dumbbells. I started with 5-pound weights and worked up to 10 pounds and 20 pounds too! The great thing about this form of exercise is that you're still burning calories long after you finish your workout. Try to get in these sessions a few times a week, even if it's just following a video at home for 20 minutes.

6. **Sexy time for you.** Whether you have a partner or not, a sexual release can be liberating. Not only does it relieve stress, it also makes you feel better. Don't be afraid to reach out and touch…yourself. I honestly

think this was my secret weapon to getting fitter.

7.   **Make sustainable changes.** If you can live the rest of your life without bread, more power to you! But if you're anything like me, you'll probably find more joy with learning the art of moderation. I still slip up sometimes, reaching for that next slice of pizza but I give myself grace. Tomorrow is a new day.

I eventually got into such amazing shape that I didn't need to wear shapewear anymore to feel good in my clothes. And when swimsuit season rolled around, I walked on the beach, letting the sun kiss my skin, feeling more confident than I had in years. I found myself oddly grateful for that awful backache that sent me to the doctor in the first place.

CHAPTER FIVE
Changes Down There: Loss Sex Drive And Vaginal Dryness, Oh My!

I can remember being a virgin my freshman year in college and feeling like the odd woman out. My friends had stories of wild sexcapades with cute boys and even not-so-cute ones. The girl who was the most experienced among us warned me, "It's a good thing you haven't done 'it' yet because once you start, you won't be able to stop."

Even though I was not waiting for marriage, I still wanted my first time be special with someone I truly loved. I had a zillion fantasies about how amazing it was going to feel and how the very act would transform my entire being. Little did I know…

I was almost 20 years old the night I lost my virginity. My boyfriend was 24 and the most handsome man I'd ever dated. His deep-set eyes, chiseled facial features and muscular frame had me under a spell. He poured me a glass of wine while soft music played. He touched me gently and savored my body, kissing my breasts and working his way down to my inner thighs. That was the first time for everything that night.

Despite my attraction to him, the act of sex was very uncomfortable.

Lucky for me, he didn't last but a few minutes. I was relieved when he finally climbed off my shell-shocked body. I'd hoped for some sweet pillow talk afterwards, but my boyfriend drifted off to sleep. I stared up at the beige ceiling. Is this what everybody is so obsessed with, I wondered.

After a few more times, I slowly adjusted to the sensation of intercourse. After a dozen times, something surprising happened, I actually started to like it. And a few months later, I found myself loving it!

Unfortunately, I did not maintain healthy boundaries with him. We started off using condoms and then he pleaded to "feel me." I gave in. Soon afterwards, my period came late which had never happened before. Hours later, I stood in the aisle of a pharmacy searching for the cheapest pregnancy test, knowing there was no way I could afford to bring a child into the world.

My negative result was the biggest relief of my life up until then. But my boyfriend ended up getting another girl pregnant while we were still together. Of course we broke up, but I promised myself that I never wanted to be in that position again.

I got on birth control pills *and* made my lovers wear condoms. As a single woman in my 20's, dating was a sizzling hot adventure. Each experience unlocked something new about my sexuality. I learned what I didn't like…no nipple biting! And I discovered that the right kiss in the right spot could deliver me to ecstasy.

By the time I met my husband, I considered myself a sexually confident, sex positive, borderline slutty. And I made no apologies about asking for what I wanted in the bedroom. That seemed to turn him on. Everything between the sheets was magic at first.

But the realities of life took a toll on my sex life. Even before perimenopause, I struggled in my marriage, and this made my libido plunge. It was impossible to get in the mood when I was working two jobs, and he could barely keep one. And I never had cookie on the brain when there was a screaming toddler who demanded all of my attention and then some.

By the time perimenopause hit me, I was resigned to living the rest of my days without sex. Nothing about it interested me at all. And I wasn't even aware of the hormonal changes going on inside my body at the time. All I felt with numbness.

On the rare occasion that Carter and I did have sex, I suffered from vaginal dryness. The discomfort always took me out of the moment to say the least. Even the fanciest lube had its limitations. If I had been more in tune with my body, I would have realized that perimenopause had played a role in this also.

As women, we are often silenced about our sexual discomfort. Even worse, societal pressures can project the narrative that intimacy is all about the man's pleasure...his orgasm is the marker of good sex and nothing else matters. That's probably why there are so many commercials on TV for erectile dysfunction and I can't recall one about a pill to help get things flowing down there for us.

To help with vaginal dryness, I searched for different solutions. When I tried soy milk, I was surprised that half a cup a day made me feel more like my old self again. Another thing that helped was raspberry tea. But the thing that played the biggest role in restoring my sexy was when I pushed the limits of my marital vowels…

One day, I was at my computer about to buy something online that I couldn't afford and I accidently clicked on a link to an adult chat website. I landed on the login page and paused. I stared at the screen.

There was an option to join the room as a guest. I hesitated. What if it was some sophisticated phishing operation to hack all my personal data? And what business did I have going to a sleazy site like that at all? But curiosity tugged at me. I made up a fake name and clicked the button to enter the room.

Right away, I was embarrassed to see the nature of the group conversation. "Hot MILF looking for a young stud to clear my pipes." "Older man seeking sugarbaby for anal arrangement." "Horny married man needs to blow his load in a thirsty mouth."

I was so overwhelmed and disgusted that I wanted to log out of the room and never look back, but then it happened. HandsomeSingleDad43 sent me a private message that simply said, "Hi."

I typed back, "Hello."

"A/S/L?"

"What?"

"Age Sex Location?"

"Sorry. I didn't know what that meant. I'm new to this."

I couldn't tell the truth and why should I? This online persona offered me the chance to be whatever I wanted to be. My heart raced as I heard my husband's footsteps on the other side of the door but that was a big part of the thrill as I kept typing:

"31 Female Pennsylvania."

I was really thirty-eight at the time and I had never lived in or near Pennsylvania. The only truth was that I was female. But chatting with a complete stranger who I couldn't even see started to make me feel more feminine and alive than I had in years.

"39 Male Florida. What's your name?"

I thought of something sexy and something that was not remotely close to my actual name. I remembered a soap opera character from years ago. "Brooke and you?"

"Vince. What brings you here tonight?"

Just then, Carter yelled out, "Have you seen my gray and blue socks?"

"In the drawer, under the…under the…" I bit my lip. Maybe I wasn't as good at multitasking as I thought.

"Got it. Thanks," he said from the next room.

I turned my attention back to Vince and saw a new message appear from him: "You still there?"

"Yes. Sorry about that."

"Good. I thought I lost you. So why did you come to this crazy place?"

"It is crazy alright. This is my first time here. I don't even know why I clicked on this chat room. What about you?"

"Bored, I guess. My kids are with my ex this weekend."

I didn't know what to say to comfort him. But I felt bad for Vince, if that was his actual name. Divorce can be ugly, especially when there are kids involved.

He broke the lull in our conversation with: "May I ask what you look like?"

I smiled to myself. He couldn't see me. I was free to give myself supermodel looks, worthy of a red-carpet strut. But I decided not to embellish too much: "I have brown eyes and dark brown hair. I'm 5'5" and curvy. People say I have a nice smile."

"You sound gorgeous, and I love a woman with curves."

"Really? Thanks."

"Do you want to know what I look like?"

"Sure."

"6'1, blue eyes and black hair. I'm in good shape because I work in construction. By the way, I'm Italian."

I blushed. He sounded so hot that I wanted to climb through the computer and see for myself. Suddenly, it happened. My inner thighs got moist at the mere thought of Vince.

"You still there, Brooke?"

"Yes! I'm right here."

"To be honest, I'm not much of a typer. Can we talk on the phone?"

"I can't right now."

"I understand but if I give you my number will you call me when you're free?"

"I'm married Vince."

"I just want to talk. We don't have to do anything you don't want to do."

"I don't know."

"My number is 813-555-3219. It's all up to you, Brooke."

I felt guilty about chatting with this strange man online. I felt even guiltier about the fact that he had awakened a desire inside of me that I thought had completely faded. But despite or, perhaps because of this, I scribbled down Vince's number on a piece of paper. I folded it up until it was no bigger than the tip of my thumb and hid it inside of an old purse.

Days passed. I was surprised how much Vince crossed my mind. I could be in the middle of doing laundry or staring at a pile of paperwork at my desk and suddenly, he was all I could think about. I wondered if he was thinking of me too.

One Saturday afternoon, Carter took Justin to run some errands and I found myself home alone. I wanted to call Vince but I thought that might be too bold. On top of that, what if he was some weirdo? I downloaded an app to create a fake phone number to disguise my own. Then, I sent him a text: "Hey."

A few minutes passed. I began to wonder if the app was faulty or if he was simply ignoring me. Then, I saw his reply: "Who's this?"

"Brooke."

";)"

":)"

"Can you talk?"

I hesitated. Then, I thought what the hell? "Okay."

I carefully clicked around on the app to make sure I called him from the fake number. He answered with a deep voice and a very distinct New Jersey accent. "Hello? Brooke?"

"Yeah, it's me." It felt strange answering to someone else's name. "I thought you were from Florida but you sound like you're from–"

"I moved down to Tampa a few years back. I'm from Hackensack, New Jersey, originally. What part of Pennsylvania did you say you were from?"

I didn't even know any cities there except: "Philadelphia."

"Oh, that's cool. I love the Phillies. My whole family are Mets fans but I can't stand 'em."

I laughed. It felt like a first date conversation. My heart pounded.

"So what are you up to?"

"My husband just went out with my son so I'm about to get dinner going. What about you?"

"My kids are with my ex again this weekend. I was putting some shelves together in the garage earlier, but I sure wish you could make me some dinner. I bet you're a great cook."

"I try." I giggled.

"Brooke, I really hope you don't take this the wrong way, but you sound so sexy."

"Thanks, I guess."

"Something about your voice really does it for me. You said you're alone, right?"

"Ah...yeah..."

"Could ya do me a favor, go in your room and get in your bed for me?"

"What?"

"Come on, it'll be fun. I'm gonna do the same thing..."

I felt a burst of wetness between my thighs as I blindly obeyed Vince. I locked my bedroom door behind me and kept my voice low. My breathing grew heavy as my mind conjured up what was going to happen next.

"Can you touch your tits for me, Brooke?"

I reached under my bra and played with my nipples. I let out a moan.

"If I was there, I'd be licking them all over."

I closed my eyes imagining Vince.

"I'm so hard for you Brooke, you have no idea… You gonna open your legs for me?"

"Yeah!" I panted.

As our steamy conversation continued, I couldn't help but touch myself everywhere. Vince's voice brought me to one of the best orgasms of my life. When it was over, I felt jubilation followed by sadness. Why couldn't I feel that way with my husband anymore? Did that count as cheating?

When I reflect back on what happened, the key to getting back in touch with my sexual side was much bigger than Vince. He was merely the vessel to come out of my fog. And ultimately, I ended up crossing more and more lines that a married woman should try to avoid. Nonetheless, it was an honest part of my journey to feel like a complete woman again.

<u>Things That Help Improve Vaginal Health and Sex Drive:</u>

1.   **Don't use heavy soap down there.** Strong soaps can have a drying effect. I once had a female doctor who told me that women should never use soap on their vaginas because it's self-cleaning. I wasn't quite comfortable with going soap-free but I switched to something very mild and only washed the outer area, never letting soap go near my vaginal canal.

2.   **Wear unsexy underwear.** When I was much younger, I had a collection of lacy panties and thongs. In retrospect, these probably put me at higher risk for infections. As I got older, I found that cotton granny panties were my friend.

3.   **Try natural lubricants.** Soy milk in moderation

can be helpful along with raspberry tea. Coconut oil can be a great natural lubricant for the vaginal area but this only works if you're not using a condom because the oils can cause latex to break down.

4.   **Touch yourself.** If more women masturbated, the world would be a happier place. Whether it's a gentle rub on your clit in the shower or you decide to buy sex toys, explore what works for you and your body. Enjoy your sexuality. You deserve it!

5.   **Eat plenty of fruits and vegetables.** Don't go on a crazy diet that restricts these. It's bad for your overall health and your lady parts will be very angry with you.

6.   **Do kegels!** This helps reduce incontinence and makes sex even better. The best thing is that it's an exercise you can do anytime, anywhere without anyone knowing. Kegels should be every woman's sexy little secret.

7.   **Get out of your comfort zone.** If you're married, this doesn't mean having an affair but don't allow yourself to become invisible as a woman. If someone pays you a compliment on your looks or how you're dressed, receive it. Glow in it. I think every woman needs reminders that they are desirable, ideally from their significant other, but let's be honest, that isn't always the case.

8.   **Try something new in the bedroom.** If you have a healthy relationship with your partner, mix things up. Whether it's a new position or having sex in a different location, you might find yourself super

turned on by the newness of it all.

9. **Be patient with your body.** Perimenopause brings about so many changes. Getting older in general brings about an even longer list. Stop comparing your body to what it used to look like in your 20's and all of the crazy acrobatic poses you could do in the bedroom once upon a dream. Embrace the now.

Once I implemented all these things, over time I began to have the best sex of my life. And sometimes, that was just by myself, and for me, that was completely fine. I went from being sexually frustrated to fully appreciating my womanhood in ways I thought were impossible. It all started by me deciding that my sex life was not over. And now, I look forward to decades of lovin' to come! Pun intended.

CHAPTER SIX
More Changes, Losing My Hair, Losing My Mind, Adult Acne, Cellulite and More

I have always had a love-hate relationship with my hair. My curls have a mind all their own, especially when humidity is introduced to the equation. Simply blow drying my hair is almost equivalent to an intense tricep workout. I have done just about everything to my precious mane…color rinses, highlights, permanent dyes, chemical straighteners, hair extensions, and shaving off the back half. And no matter what I did, my curls would grow back, stronger and more determined than ever. Until the day they didn't.

Around the time I turned thirty-eight, I distinctly remember shedding more hair on my brushes and combs than usual. And on wash days, there was always more to pluck out of the drain stopper. But I ignored all of these signs until the morning I went to style my hair as usual and it was so limp and thin that I barely recognized myself.

I assumed that my hair loss was due to stress. And that was definitely a part of the equation, but looking back, this was also an early sign of perimenopause. At the time, I didn't have any tools to combat this, so I grabbed my ponytail holder and rushed out the door.

The other thing that I started to notice was facial hair. A dark strand sprung up in the middle of my chin, announcing its presence to the world. It was soon joined by another and another. The three "beard" kateers challenged my femininity. Was I going to have to start shaving now?

And it got even stranger. One day, I was in the shower about to do a self-exam on my breasts and I saw a hair near my nipple. *What?!* It couldn't be. All this time, maybe I wasn't a woman at all. Perhaps, I was secretly a sasquatch. I reasoned that the only upside to this was that I could quit my lousy job and join the circus already.

Around then, I was shocked to see yet another change. Pimples! And for me, they were big, red, and juicy. It was a throwback to one of the things I hated most about my teenage years. And unfortunately, my attempts to dry them out with a dab of toothpaste fell flat.

I couldn't help but laugh at the irony of it all. Wrinkles were coming in accompanied by adult acne. Good foundation was my only salvation. But every night, when I removed my makeup, I was confronted with the reality of what was underneath.

Another thing that I could not ignore was more pronounced cellulite, especially on my thighs. And cutting back on fried foods did not move the needle on this. I can still remember seeing my mother get dressed as a child and how she described hers as "cottage cheese." She flashed a teasing smile but there was a sense of shame buried in her laughter. I went from wondering if there was a way to reverse my cellulite to wondering if it was going to get worse with the passing years.

It turns out that hormonal changes during perimenopause can cause loss of hair on the top of your head and the appearance of it in places that might surprise and embarrass you. Our bodies are a delicate balance of estrogen, testosterone, and progesterone. These all shift around as women hit middle age.

Some of the symptoms I experienced were probably more pronounced because I had recently stopped taking the pill. Many women claim that birth control can make the transition to perimenopause easier because it helps to balance out hormones. Everyone has to make the choice that is right for their bodies and consult with a doctor.

For me personally, I didn't want to take the pill anymore because I was hardly having sex and I had been on it for so many years that I wanted to get to know my body again naturally. While I wasn't fully prepared for the tsunami of things that happened in the aftermath, I did find a way to cope with my symptoms.

I'd read a lot about the benefits of red wine for the skin, the antioxidants in particular. And as a lover of wine, I was all for that. I started drinking a glass or two of a cabernet and I also made a habit of actually putting the wine directly on my acne and blemishes. I also stopped wearing foundation every day and reached for the sunscreen instead. Within a few weeks, I saw a significant improvement in my complexion.

The day I went to see my general practitioner with concerns about perimenopause, he seemed more alarmed by my facial hair than all the other symptoms I described. He wanted to give me a referral for electrolysis, but I declined. I decided to buy a facial hair remover at the pharmacy and in less than 30 seconds, the strands of hair on my chin and nipples were gone. Problem solved!

For the thinning hair on my head, I tried things like thickening shampoos and deep conditioners. I even did some wild stuff like hair masks made of eggs and mayonnaise. What a waste of groceries! My hair was just as thin as ever and it smelled like rotting potato salad.

One thing that did help a bit with my hair was to embrace its natural texture and color. I decided to stop all of the constant blow drying and give the highlights a rest. I feel that this was the break my hair needed because within a few months, it was in much better shape. The thickness was not fully restored but I celebrated the noticeable improvement.

When I wanted to snap into a sexy look without damaging my fragile curls, I popped on a cute wig. It was a fun way to transform my look and I bought a few for variety. Much to my surprise, strangers couldn't even tell the difference. And even if they could, I didn't care.

As for my cellulite, I began to make peace with the fact that it wasn't going anywhere. Some statistics indicate that 90% of women have some form of it. I figured why should I be ashamed of it? So what, I didn't have the body of a teenager anymore? But if I'm being completely honest, I spent a lot of time picking apart my body back then too!

As women, we are often told directly or indirectly that our value is tethered to our appearance. If you're not deemed as "beautiful" then you're not worth much. But even the most gorgeous women might find themselves in a loop of self-consciousness and worthlessness.

I wanted to break free of that for myself. So I am that woman with thick thighs and cellulite who you might see in the summertime with a pair of short-shorts because why the hell not? And when I make love, I am of the mindset that we can absolutely keep the lights on!

I've got nothing to hide and what good would it do anyway? He's gonna see it all. And now, I've built myself up to a point where I want him to. If for some reason, he's not into the "real" me then it does neither one of us any good for me to pretend to be something I ain't.

I also made a better effort to stop being so judgmental of other women's looks too. Even at my heaviest, I was quick to glance over at some chick I didn't even know and label her as "fat." Or there are many times when I used to walk by someone and wonder, *Why on earth is she wearing that?* Well, frankly it's none of my business and I don't want it to be anymore.

Just existing as a woman is hard enough without all the constant whispers about who's beautiful and who's hideous. I strive to live my life without obsessing over that stuff and I hope any woman who reads this follows suit. Let's face it, at the end of the day, many of us are competing for men who may or may not even shower every day. And don't even get me started on how many of them never heard of "manscaping."

Speaking of hair down there…I recently got my first gray pubic hair. I guess that is a true mark of maturity if there ever was one! At first, I used to shave constantly, desperate to make it invisible, but now, I'm a lot more relaxed. Any man I deem special enough to see the most intimate part of me should not be bothered with it. And if he is, then he's not the man for me.

As you may have surmised, I am no longer married to Carter. I will delve deeper into what happened in the next chapter, which is all about relationships. And navigating dating as a woman over forty can be challenging. But the truth is that it's no cakewalk for anyone. I think the thing that has helped me form genuine connections with the opposite sex is being my authentic self.

And speaking of authenticity, I no longer lie about my age. The craziest thing is that I actually look younger than I did when my perimenopause symptoms first began at the age of thirty-six. But I take pride in looking people in the eye and telling them the real number. I feel that I have earned every single year. Also, when you lie about your age, you have to come up with a string of other lies to maintain the facade. I am too busy living a full life to go down that road ever again.

Now as I approach my forty-third birthday, I am proud to have the smoothest skin I ever had and the most body confidence I've ever had. When I look in the mirror, I am no longer picking myself apart. Even on the days my hair refuses to cooperate! Instead of cursing at the ceiling, I smile, reminding myself I'm lucky that I still have some strands of my own. And a cute wig is always within arm's reach too!

<u>Tips for hair loss, adult acne, cellulite and more:</u>

1.   **Drink enough water.** This will help with your skin, hair, and bodily functions. Dehydration only worsens the symptoms of perimenopause. While it might not be necessary to drink eight glasses a day, drink enough so that your urine is clear and doesn't

smell rank. I'm not trying to be gross, just honest here!

2.   **Red wine in moderation can help.** Even if you're not a wine drinker, you can dab a bit of dry red wine on your skin. For me, this was a game changer. And in my case, having a glass with dinner was the icing on the cake.

3.   **Eat more protein.** Your body needs plenty of protein for fuel. It also helps your hair, skin, and nails. One easy way to add some into your day is to put a spoonful of collagen in your morning coffee and reach for the yogurt instead of the donut. Simple changes can lead to significant results.

4.   **Minimize stress.** Perimenopause can cause hair loss. But oftentimes, stress is an even bigger factor. Go for walks, meditate, pray, and make sure you find time to laugh out loud. Your body and your hair will thank you!

5.   **HIIT exercise to burn fat.** If you want to burn more fat to help reduce the appearance of cellulite, High Intensity Interval Training is your friend. Ease into this because this is a very intense workout but it can be a game changer.

6.   **Embrace your natural hair.** Air drying instead of blow drying and cutting back on dyes and chemicals can help a lot when it comes to thinning hair. Yes, I have some grays that show, and my curls still have a mind of their own. But that's fine with me. Maybe it's fine with you too.

7.   **Wigs and hats.** A collection of cool wigs and hats can be awesome. But be sure to always take care

of your real hair underneath and wear the appropriate wig caps. Also, this is a very bad idea on steamy summer days, your scalp feeling like it's on fire combined with a possible hot flash ain't cute.

8. **Love your body.** For me personally, I started to feel much better about myself when I stopped comparing my body to the airbrushed beauties online and on TV. Besides, they don't even look like that. Loving your body is all about being grateful for who you are and your life in general.

By doing these things, my perimenopause journey became a lot easier. I was no longer fighting to look like I used to. That woman is gone. But what remains is still amazing, at least I'd like to think so!

CHAPTER SEVEN
Relationship Changes, Redefining What Love and Life Looks Like

Like many women, I was raised and conditioned to always be polite. And this went beyond table manners or saying "please" and "thank you." From the time I was a little girl, I watched the women around me repress their true opinions and keep complaints to a minimum. My mother always stressed, "Nobody wants to be around a 'Debbie Downer' or a 'Negative Nancy.'"

There were times when I took this to the extreme. Like… eating Aunt Blair's golden raisin cookies that upset my stomach simply because I didn't want to hurt her feelings. And without fail, she'd bake a new batch every time I came to visit. Her eyes lit up when I took a bite and forced myself to grin, all the while, a tornado of gas formed inside me.

"I made these just for you, honey," she'd say. "I know they're your favorite. Be sure and take some home now."

Even in my 20's when I was single and independent, I found myself reluctant to open up to a man I dated about what really turned me on. Instead, I became the E.G.O.T. of faking orgasms all in an effort to *please* him. When I think back on it now, all of that panting and hollering was pitiful. Why didn't I just pipe up and say, "Hey, I like this instead of that or can we try this…"

Being conflict-avoidant has always been my comfort zone. But perimenopause snapped me right out of that. I didn't have the energy to pretend everything was okay *and* deal with all the changes happening to my body as I approached middle age. I had to be honest with myself and everyone around me for the first time in my life. It was uncomfortable and painful, but ultimately liberating.

The first thing I had to do was take inventory of my whole life. My marriage. My job. My parenting. My relationships with family members and friends. I can distinctly remember writing a list of all the things I wanted and *needed* to be different. I was scared but the thought of politely remaining in silence terrified me even more.

I began with what I knew was going to be the most difficult task. Carter. Through all the rough times we had, there was still love underneath it all. But I was so exhausted and frustrated by the time I started to open up about my true feelings that I'd already checked out of the marriage.

I told him that I needed us to get our financial house in order. I needed him to work a job consistently and build a career. I needed us to communicate better about decisions both big and small. Carter had a habit of buying on impulse and there was a revolving door of his family members who used to just pop-up without much notice. I just couldn't do it anymore.

His reaction was to call me selfish and yell that I didn't

really love him or his family. He became so defensive I didn't even recognize him as the man I'd fallen in love with all those years ago. Our shouting matches escalated. On one night in particular where he called me vile names and glared at me with contempt. He banged his fists on the wall and I cowered, bracing for him to hit me. The whole time, I hoped our son in the next room could not hear what was going on but I was sure he did. That's when I knew I couldn't stay in my marriage anymore.

Most of the times when a couple separates, it's usually the man who moves out. But Carter refused to leave so I knew I'd have to find my own place. The thought of leaving the comfort of our suburban home which literally had a white picket fence was hard to wrap my head around. But staying there with him was no longer an option.

I found a small apartment in a noisy part of town near a warehouse district. The place was so barebones that it didn't have air conditioning or a washer and dryer unit. Nonetheless, it was the fresh start my soul so desperately needed. And even with all the chaos outside my window, I got some of the best sleep of my life.

The hardest thing about leaving Carter was the strain it put on our son. But we were able to work out a visitation schedule where we both agreed to equal time with him. In my crowded little apartment, I tried to shower as much love on Justin as possible. We cooked, read together and watched cartoons that made us laugh out loud.

He often asked me why I left Daddy and I explained to him in the calmest voice I could muster, "Sometimes two people get married and love each other and things change. But the one thing that will never change is that we both love you." Then, I gave him a big hug and kissed his forehead.

On the days when Carter wasn't there, I found myself with something I hadn't had in years…"me time." It was odd at first. But soon, I leaned into the opportunity to rediscover the person I was. I read a ton of books, went for long walks, and reflected deeply about what I wanted the next season of my life to look like.

At the time, I was still working two jobs. But eventually, I found one job that paid enough for me to cover my bills. Unfortunately, since Carter's income was sporadic, there was no hope for spousal or child support or anything like that. I was completely on my own.

Don't get me wrong, I was much happier, but there were days when I struggled. Putting in an eight-hour shift, sometimes nine-hours, started to take more of a toll on me. I knew that perimenopause and menopause could intensify an already challenging workplace environment. I decided that I wanted to make bigger career changes.

I set a goal for myself that I didn't want to retire from a "day job." But beyond that, I wanted to do something that brought me more joy than staring at spreadsheets and churning out analytic reports. I'd always been passionate about writing, so I decided to take a few classes online.

Eventually, I started to write and publish books under a pen name. Over time, I also got hired as a ghostwriter for other people. It was a fun, creative outlet and it enabled me to supplement my income. Although I don't make enough to quit my day job, I am grateful I took the first step.

The timing could not have worked out better because

things got more stressful at the office than ever before. It felt good to know that I had different ways to bring in much needed money and my confidence and bank accounts grew. Eventually, I want to transition to publishing books full-time so I'm actively looking for ways to realize that goal.

Of all the books I've written, this has been the most therapeutic by far. It is my sincerest hope that it does provide a blueprint for other women who find themselves in similar situations. By no means am I suggesting that you blow up your whole life and walk away from your marriage, but on the other hand, I am also living proof that if that is a decision you make, you can come out on the other side stronger, more resilient and more at peace.

I'm sure you're also wondering about my current dating life and what it's been like. As a divorced single mother, I was very reluctant to get into a new relationship with just anyone. But I welcomed the opportunity to just have fun and date. It was nice to put on a cute outfit and try new restaurants. Of course Prince Charming wasn't always sitting across from me at the table. But to my surprise, I did make a genuine connection to a wonderful man whom we will call Kyle for the sake of this book.

I was drawn to him from the start. He was handsome and fit with a great smile and captivating eyes. He was also six years younger, so I assumed that he wasn't looking for anything serious. And that was just fine with me.

From our very first kiss, the chemistry was amazing. But I was still determined to keep my cool. I didn't blow up his phone or ruminate over every text message exchange. I had way too much going on in my life for any of that. I think my laid-back approach drew him closer. He was more accustomed to women becoming obsessed with him, and overtime, I came to understand why. He was the whole package and then some.

On top of being a good listener with a kind heart, Kyle was also super supportive. If my sink was broken, he'd be right there to fix it. If I was stressed, his strong hands were on standby for a massage. And if I was drowning in bills, he'd help out.

I felt very fortunate to have him in my life, but I still wanted to take my time when it came to introducing him to Justin. But soon things became more serious between us and we fell in love. It was unexpected in the most amazing way.

In an era where online podcasters and articles highlight all the flaws of women over forty, especially single mothers, it's refreshing to experience a relationship with someone who appreciates my value. What I share with Kyle is the adventure my heart had always been longing for. And I can't wait to see what's next on our horizon.

When it came to my relationship with family members and friends, I also put up more boundaries to avoid burnout. For example, instead of driving all across town to visit with various relatives, I would ask if everyone could meet up at one house instead. There were times when I got pushback, but I refused to let it phase me anymore. I was determined to find ways to take out as many stress points in my life as possible.

I also got a million times better at saying "No." And sometimes, "Hell no!" I became the most authentic version of myself. Some people were less than thrilled about the changes I made but I couldn't live solely for their comfort. I am disappointed in myself that it took perimenopause to get to this point.

In many online message boards about perimenopause, husbands complain about their wives being very irritable and having a short fuse. Hormonal changes can impact these things, but I can't help but think it is also a culmination of years of the same "politeness" that I desperately tried to up-hold. I am relieved that I gave myself permission to be a full human being who isn't afraid to label her emotions or express sadness, disappointment, or anger. But for the record, I still say "please" and "thank you."

<u>Tips for navigating perimenopause with loved ones:</u>

1.   **Talk to them honestly about the life change.** This conversation should go beyond a list of symp-toms and jokes about hot flashes. You need to help the person understand what perimenopause is and exact-ly how it is impacting your health: physically, mental-ly, and emotionally. In many cases, it might be a good idea to share articles, books, or other resources with your loved one for clarity, especially if it's a man.

2.   **Speak up for yourself.** Do not silence your voice or your true feelings. If someone lets you down, pull them aside and express your thoughts as soon as possible. If they continue to let you down, try to put some distance between the two of you if at all possible. Toxic people will only pile on more stress and sleepless nights.

3.   **Make your life as comfortable as possible.**

Whether it's an extreme change like divorce or a simple adjustment like repainting your room a brighter color, you deserve peace. No human should have to live without it. Don't convince yourself that you have to suffer for anyone. Once again, you deserve peace. And your body, mind and spirit will thank you for it.

4.   **Just say no.** If you don't feel up to running that extra errand or baking brownies for the school's fundraiser, you don't have to. If your teenager asks for another dog and you're already overwhelmed with the pets you have, then let them know it's not the right time. Often our fear of disappointing others can paint us into a corner. You must stop worrying about them. Take yourself off the bottom of your priority list. And make a promise to yourself not to end up there ever again.

5.   **Claim your happiness.** Plan that dream vacation. Even if you can't afford it now, start putting away a bit every month until you're on your way to Paris or the place of your dreams. Sing your favorite song out loud. Treat yourself to something special. Love the woman you are. You will find that your happiness translates to all the people who love you. On the other hand, the people who make you feel bad about setting boundaries are pretenders who never had your best intentions at heart.

Of all the things I did to help cope with perimenopause, these were the hardest to tackle. It was a lot easier to cut back on desserts than to make big and broad changes to my entire world. But I had to decide if I was going to merely be alive and remain a body drawing breath or take the plunge and live this amazing, unpredictable, exciting, and worthwhile thing known as *life*. I never dreamed I would be this happy and I wish all of that for you and more. I hope you got something of value out of this book. Thank you for taking this journey with me.

FREE RESOURCES TO HELP:

Weight Loss/Management:
Lose It! App (Available on Android and iPhone)

There is a free version that allows you to track calories, macros, sodium and sugar intake everyday. You can also log exercise. I never upgraded to the paid account, this was all I needed to get on the right track and stay there.

Exercise Tutorial:
Melissa Neill's Channel (Available on YouTube)

There are many fitness channels on YouTube but I especially love Melissa because she speaks from personal experience about her journey all the way through post-menopause. Her exercises are easy to follow and you don't have to buy expensive gym equipment. After you master the basics, you can work your way up to more complex routines. She is a true inspiration for wellness and overall fitness.

Better Sleep:
Brown Noise | 12 hrs - (Available on Spotify)

I tried different sounds and apps and this was my absolute favorite. I get a very good night's sleep and I love that it plays for 12 hours. If I do wake up in the middle of the night, it is much easier to fall back asleep with this on.

Sexy Time:
Chat-Avenue - (Available Online)

There are several free chat rooms and a lot of excitement to be found. This is also where I met Vince. Always be safe online and I suggest remaining annoymous as I did.